MW00512405

Heal your Gut Cookbook

Delicious & Nourishing Recipes for Stages 1 to 6 to Feel Great and Lose Weight

Abigail Kahn

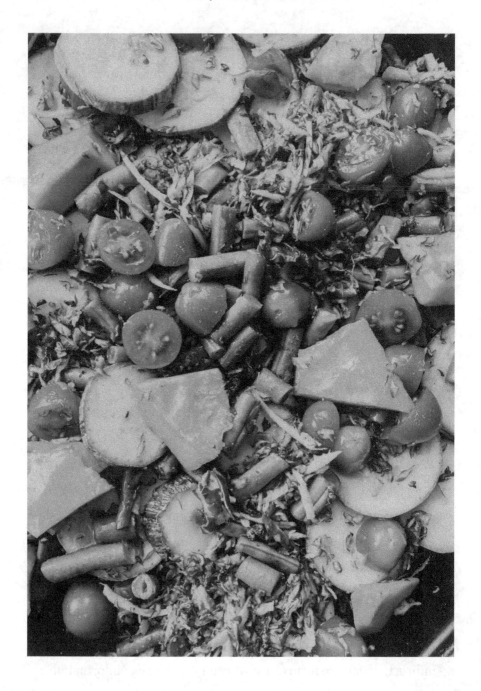

Table of Contents

INTRODUCTION 8

CHAPTER 1: THE GUT AND PSYCHOLOGY SYNDRO....................................12

    CAUSES OF GAPS 14

CHAPTER 2: THE GAPS DIET..18

    DIFFERENT STAGES OF GAP DIET 20

    INTRODUCTION DIET: STAGE 1 21

    STAGE 2.. 24

    STAGE 3.. 25

    STAGE 4.. 25

    STAGE 5.. 26

    STAGE 6.. 27

CHAPTER 3: FOOD TO EAT AND TO AVOID 28

    BENEFITS OF GAPS DIET.. 32

    SPRING CLEAN YOUR BODY WITH THE GAPS DIET!.................................... 32

    HOW DOES THE GAPS DIET HELP WITH IBS? 33

    HOW DOES THE GAP DIET AFFECT CONSTIPATION, HERE'S THE TRUTH?.................. 35

CHAPTER 4: SUPPLEMENTATION 38

    DEGLYCYRRHIZINATED LICORICE 38

    BETAINE HYDROCHLORIC ACID 38

    L-GLUTAMINE.. 39

    SLIPPERY ELM.. 40

    DIGESTIVE ENZYMES 40

    ALOE VERA.. 41

CHAPTER 5: BREAKFAST RECIPE..42

1.   MANGO GREEN TEA SHAKE..42

2.   MINTY PAPAYA SMOOTHIE...44

3.   COCOA BANANA PROTEIN POWER..46

4.   SLOW-COOKED PEPPERS FRITTATA...48

5.   VEGGIE BOWLS..50

6.   SIMPLE STEEL CUTS...52

7.   VANILLA FLAVORED OATS...54

8.   FETA BAKED EGGS 56

9.   BUCKWHEAT PORRIDGE..58

CHAPTER 6: SNACK RECIPES..60

10. CREAMY BUTTERNUT PORRIDGE 60

11. AVOCADO AND SAUERKRAUT 61

12. ONION EGG SCRAMBLE..62

13. LACTO-FERMENTED CARROTS..63

14. ALMOND CAKE 65

15. INSTANT BANANA PUDDING..67

16. CHOCOLATE-ORANGE-RASPBERRY CUPCAKES..................................69

17. CHOCOLATE-ORANGE-RASPBERRY FROSTING...................................71

18. GRAHAM CRACKERS..73

CHAPTER 7: LUNCH RECIPES 76

19. AVOCADO SALMON SALAD...76

20. CHICKEN TACO SALAD...77

21. AFRICAN CHICKEN PEANUT STEW..79

22. HAWAIIAN TOASTIE...81

23. CHICKEN ALFREDO PASTA BAKE...83

24. LAMB DEAL..86

25. BAKED BEEF CASSEROLE 88

26. CARROT BAKED CHICKEN 90

CHAPTER 8: DINNER RECIPES 92

27.   BAKED LEMON-BUTTER FISH 92

28.   FISH TACO BOWL 94

29.   SCALLOPS WITH CREAMY BACON SAUCE 96

30.   BEEF STEW 98

31.   IRISH STEW 100

32.   LINGUINE AND BRUSSELS SPROUTS 102

33.   RUSTIC VEGETABLE AND BROWN RICE BOWL 104

34.   ROASTED BRUSSELS SPROUTS AND PECANS 106

CHAPTER 9: SOUP AND SALAD RECIPES 108

35.   CARROT SOUP 108

36.   CELERY SOUP 110

37.   CREAMY SALMON DILL SALAD 112

38.   BROCCOLI SOUP 114

39.   GARDEN SALAD WITH ORANGES AND OLIVES 115

40.   LEMONY LENTIL SALAD WITH SALMON 117

41.   RAW WINTER PERSIMMON SALAD 119

42.   TABBOULEH- ARABIAN SALAD 121

CHAPTER 10: DESSERTS RECIPES 124

43.   WATERMELON CREAM 124

44.   GRAPES STEW 125

45.   COLD LEMON SQUARES 126

46.   CHOCOLATE CAKE WITH CHOCOLATE FROSTING 127

47.   MIXED BERRY CRUMBLE 130

48.   PEANUT BUTTER CHOCOLATE CHIP COOKIES 132

49.   STAR SUGAR COOKIES 134

50.   BROWNIES 136

CONCLUSION 138

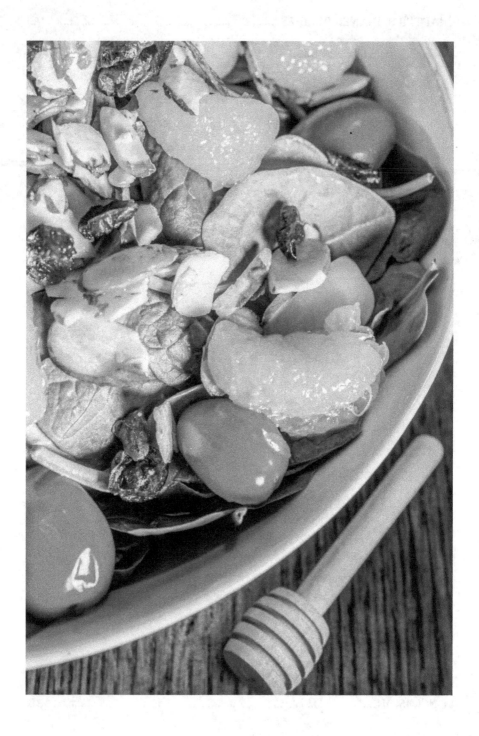

Introduction

The GAPS diet, or Gut and Psychological Syndrome diet, is based on the idea that a person should listen to his or her gut. That is, a person with Irritable Bowel Syndrome likely has extensive stomach damage. Specifically, the IBS patient probably has tears in the lining of the stomach or the "gut wall."

Because of this, he or she will have trouble digesting food and may mistake discomfort for food sensitivities or allergies that haven't existed before. The GAPS diet does include a sensitivity test for various foods, but in truth, many people who use it, especially those with IBS, just need an intense diet and lifestyle change.

By the time people are desperate enough to consider changing their eating habits, they are usually already coping with intense symptoms in themselves and/or in their children. They may also have been sleep-deprived for some time. Plus, previous attempts to remedy the issues may have all but swallowed their wallets. For all of these reasons, people coming to the GAPS program tend to be overwhelmed and stressed to the hilt.

Before starting any aspect of the program, please read this Guide in its entirety. Details about any given aspect of the program are presented throughout. To be successful on the program with the minimum of frustration, it will be important to have read this entire book through at least once before beginning. Jumping in before reading all of the material presented in this Guide may make your journey more difficult and stressful than necessary.

A damaged gut produces a lot of toxins. Items we use every day, as well as elements in our general environment, may also be toxic. As Dr. Campbell-McBride notes, the human body has a "detoxification system" that is responsible for the elimination of internal and environmental toxins. If this system is overloaded and cannot process the volume of toxins present, the toxic substances are stored in various tissues of one's body (e.g., skin, joints, and muscles). This causes symptoms. Although the diet and supplements will go far to reduce the overall toxic load, they cannot in themselves relieve the body of years of accumulated muck. Additional steps are needed. Detox supports, such as home-pressed juices, supplemented baths, and daily bowel movements, can help remove the existing load as well as any unpreventable new burdens. Conscious lifestyle choices can limit any further unnecessary exposures.

The idea behind the GAPS diet is that there is a connection between the state of a person's digestive system and the health of the rest of the body. GAPS has been known to improve many health conditions including autism, mental disorders, eating disorders, asthma, chronic fatigue syndrome, eczema, allergies, and many more. Why does what you eat impact all of these health conditions? According to Dr. Campbell it happens because processed foods and high fructose corn syrup have been destroying the natural balance of microbes in our intestinal system. The GAPS diet aims to restore us to a natural equilibrium.

To get results, you have to stay on this expensive and time-consuming diet for a minimum of six months and possibly up to as much as two years. That takes a lot of money and time, but every parent of an autistic child knows that a smile, or even just a response, is a treasure beyond all others. If the GAPS diet can help bring that about, it's wonderful. And soon, perhaps, Dr. Mulloy and other researchers will be able to establish once and for all whether this diet really does work on autism and other illnesses.

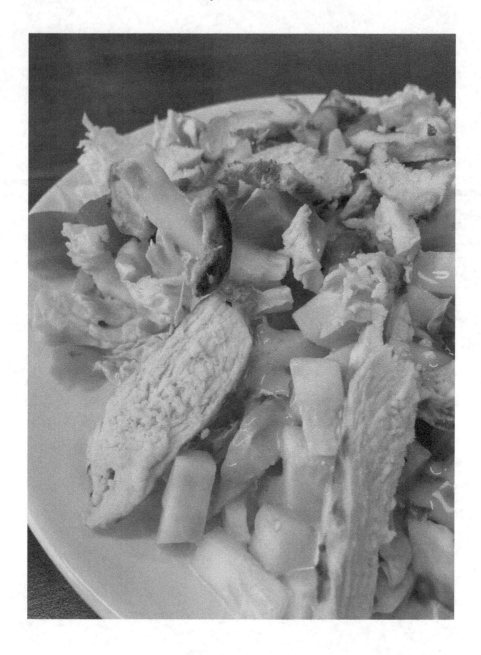

Chapter 1: The Gut and Psychology Syndro

The gastrointestinal tract is home to many tiny organisms. Most are "good," that is, they help our bodies to digest food. They also control the "bad" microbes—the ones that make toxins. When the balance between "good" and "bad" gut organisms changes, we no longer can digest and absorb food properly. Natasha says that this leads to a buildup of toxins throughout the body that contributes to a wide range of problems from learning disabilities and food allergies all the way to such things as diabetes and autoimmune disorders.

Why does this happen? She says it is because processed foods and high fructose corn syrup have been ruining the natural balance of microbes in our intestinal system. Abnormal species have taken over, releasing toxins and damaging the delicate lining of the GI tract.

The liver does help to detoxify the body, but Dr. Campbell-McBride reports that it needs assistance from us. Juices, she says, provide gentle and effective detoxification. Probiotics from supplements and fermented foods restore those helpful bacteria and yeasts that remove harmful chemicals from our systems.

Besides detoxification, she emphasizes that the most basic step is to heal the gut. Take food allergies, for example.

For many people, this internal damage has been going on for a very long time, so it can only heal slowly. Natasha reports that it can take as much as 18 months before people with serious problems, who are on the introduction to the GAPS diet, begin to see results. GAP Syndrome *can* be healed, but it is a complex as well as time-consuming process, according to Dr. Campbell-McBride.

Besides diet, she says, people also need to take these nutritional supplements:

- A therapeutic probiotic that has as many species of helpful microbes as possible in a high concentration, at least eight billion per gram
- Essential fatty acids. Natasha recommends seed/nut oil blends or fish oil
- Vitamin A, preferably in the form of cod liver oil
- Digestive enzymes in the form of betaine HCl with pepsin, as well as pancreatic enzymes
- Vitamin and mineral supplements, although not at the beginning of the GAPS Diet

Finally, to make sure Guts and Psychology Syndrome doesn't return after the diet has been completed, Natasha recommends making the right lifestyle changes to reduce exposure to environmental chemicals and other toxins. The most important thing is to watch what we eat, though. All the external changes in the world won't help very much if our GI microbial balance is disturbed and there is ongoing damage to our intestinal lining.

Before looking at the GAPS Diet, let's take a closer look at its two guiding principles: detoxification and probiotics.

Causes of GAPS

It's hard to pinpoint a single cause for a gut syndrome, but some frequent contributors often lead to disturbing the flora balance in the gut. Let's discuss some of these factors that cause ill health to your gut.

Food and Environmental Sensitivities

Food, along with environmental sensitivities may be the cause of a leaky gut syndrome. These sensitivities, likewise referred to as delayed hypersensitivity differs from real food allergies. The widespread of these sensitivities is more widely-recognized today than in previous years as around 24 percent of American adults claimed that they have food and environmental sensitivities.

Environmental Contaminants

Every day, we are exposed to numerous environmental and household chemicals which put stress on our immune defenses and breaking the body's ability to self-repair. This can lead to a chronic delay of necessary routine repairs. Our immune system pays attention to many areas at one time and those far from the digestive system are affected - connective tissues are breaking down as the body loses trace minerals like calcium, magnesium, and potassium. Toxic chemicals deplete our reserves of buffering minerals, causing acidosis in the cells and tissue and swelling in the cells.

Chronic Stress

When you are experiencing a prolonged stress, your immune system's ability to respond quickly is altered affecting your ability to heal. Every time your body feels that you are in an emergency situation and this is what happens when you are under stress, it prepares itself to be in a "fight or flight" mode and produces hormones like adrenaline to help you out of danger. However, when this often happens, there is overproduction in your adrenaline making your insulin-resistant as it goes on and on, your body loses its ability to sense danger. It can no longer tell the difference between the typical day to day stress and real stress.

Once in a real state of danger like being face to face with a vicious beast, the body reacts to such stressor by producing less secretory IgA or sIgA, one of the front lines of the body's immune defense system and lessens DHEA - an anti-aging, anti-stress adrenal hormone. It likewise slows down the digestion and peristalsis, decreases blood flow to digestive organs, and produces metabolites.

Dysbiosis

Dysbiosis is a condition wherein there is a microbial imbalance inside the body which contributes to the existence of a leaky gut. When there is an overproduction of candida, a fungus responsible for nutrient absorption and digestion when in contained comparable levels in the body, it can break down the walls of the intestine lining and penetrates into the bloodstream. Candidiasis must be taken into consideration when leaky gut is suspected. There are other parasites and microbes like salmonella, amoebas, shigella, Helicobacter, giardia, and many others that cause irritation to the intestinal lining and cause gastrointestinal symptoms. People with digestive illness or a history of it have a greater tendency to acquire leaky gut syndrome.

Overconsumption of Alcoholic Beverages

Although alcoholic drinks contain some nutrients, it takes many nutrients to metabolize. Among these are the B-complex vitamins. Alcoholic beverages contain substances that are also toxic to cells. When alcohol is metabolized in the liver, toxins are either broken down or further stored in the body. Alcohol abuse puts a strain on the liver and this affects digestive competency and further damages the intestinal tract.

Poor Food Choices

Consumption of low-fiber diet can increase the time of food digestion, allowing toxic by-products to accumulate and cause irritation in the gut mucosa. Diets of highly processed foods likewise injure the intestinal lining and they are invariably low in fiber and nutrients but contains a high level of food additives, restructured fats, and sugar. This kind of foods promotes inflammation of the Gastrointestinal (GI) tract. Therefore it is essential to know and remember that even foods that we thought of as healthful like wheat, eggs, and milk can, in fact, irritate the gut lining.

Use of Medications

There are medications such as nonsteroidal drugs like Advil, Motrin, and aspirin that can damage brush borders allowing partially digested food particles along with toxins and microbes to get into the bloodstream. Steroid drugs and birth control likewise create conditions that help feed fungi that damage the intestinal lining. Other things that can significantly disrupt the GI balance are chemotherapy medications and radiation.

Chapter 2: The gaps Diet

Many choose to stay on GAPS for many more months or years because they are enjoying it and are continuing to see improvements in their health. Once your gut has healed, chances are very high that you will be able to incorporate other quality foods, such as potatoes or sourdough bread, into your weekly diet. You will also likely be able to get away with eating anything you wish on occasion. Once strengthened, your body will be able to process and eliminate the toxins without noticeable stress. Hopefully, you will not revert back to a conventional diet because that would create toxic overload again.

What causes an imbalance of gut flora? No one thing will do it on its own. Contributing factors include diet, antibiotics, environmental toxins (e.g., lead, mercury, pollution, and chlorine), contraceptive pills, other medications, steroids, and stress. An imbalance in the pregnant mother's gut flora can affect the baby (e.g., when the child comes through the birth canal, his system is filled with an imbalance of flora), and compromised breast milk may offer limited benefits in terms of probiotics. Granted, we live in a world that includes environmental toxins and stress, and antibiotics do have their place. The GAPS program does not propose that you quit work, become a recluse, and live in a yurt (unless you want to!). It's all about your total toxic load. Select your toxins consciously and move them out regularly. For example, is it really necessary to replace your carpets this year? Is pesticide-free food an option for your family? Cleaning with vinegar and baking soda can achieve tremendous results throughout the house without putting your family at risk with harsh cleaning chemicals. Is your illness so severe that it calls for antibiotics, or will rest and ginger tea do the trick?

Regardless of the origin of one's gut imbalance, in the GAPS healing program we aim to address it by (1) sealing the gut wall, (2) rebuilding the body's natural detoxification system so that it can effectively release toxins day after day, and (3) bringing bacteria and yeasts to an optimal balance in the ideal locations for each type. GAPS recognizes that every type of bacteria and yeast has a positive role in its optimal locations and numbers. Every microbe is simply seeking its ideal conditions, as determined by acidity levels, temperature, presence of other bacteria, and so on. Through GAPS, we create in our gut the conditions in which specific bacteria thrive, while the rest stay in their optimal balance in their own ideal locations. One way in which we do this is by taking in only the types of foods even a compromised gut can quickly and thoroughly break down, leaving no remnants to act as food for microbes that would otherwise overwhelm the gut and break down the gut lining. Microbes that do not belong in the gut, or which should not exist in such high proportions there, reduce in number or completely die away from that location. However, they will continue their positive roles in the locations and/or numbers that are correct for them.

This process of balancing microbes and rebuilding the body's natural detoxification system takes time. For most people, a minimum of 18–24 months will be required. The exact timeline will be different for everyone, because it depends on one's age, degree of illness, adherence to the program, number of recommendations incorporated, and the individual body's ability to cope with detoxification. In general, a person should stay on the program for 6–12 months after the last symptom has reared its ugly head (after the initial two years, if any symptoms are persisting, one may at that point consider incorporating additional intensive therapies, such as specific chelation approaches as presented by Dr. Campbell-McBride in her FAQ document).

Different Stages of GAP diet

Each stage of the GAPS diet allows for a gradual re-introduction of different foods. Therefore, Stage 1 of the GAPS diet is the stage where you are most restricted and you will likely find it to be the most challenging. The sudden change in coming off a diet that was probably loaded with foods that did not sit well with your body can be tough and may lead to some detox symptoms where you feel intense cravings at times. The grass is truly greener on the other side, so please stick with it. The introduction diet, if done right, will keep you very well nourished and hydrated, which is exactly what your body needs during the adjustment period. To set yourself up for success, it is a good idea to prep a couple of homemade stocks ahead of time and to be prepared with lots of GAPS-approved vegetables before you get started. This way, you can grab and go, and it doesn't take ages to put your meals together. Stage 1 is a very basic diet and consists of the following foods:

Introduction Diet: Stage 1

The GAPS introduction diet focuses on nourishing foods that nourish the gut lining with things like amino acids, fats, vitamins, and minerals. The foods help to renew the gut lining. The introduction part of the GAPS diet also initially removes any fiber, as well as other substances that may cause irritation to the gut and could ultimately interfere with the healing process. Not everyone knows that they have inflammation in the gut so, by focusing on the nourishing and supporting foods, the gut is allowed to heal even in cases where inflammation has gone undetected. The GAPS introduction diet also includes probiotic-rich, healthy bacteria right from the get-go so the gut can start repairing itself and heal with beneficial bacteria.

- Pumpkin
- Winter squash
- Onion

- Garlic
- Carrots
- Broccoli
- Cauliflower
- Fermented vegetable juice
- Turnips
- Homemade stock
- Meats & fish cooked into the stock such as:
- Beef
- Lamb
- Chicken
- Turkey
- Fish
- Non-fibrous vegetables cooked in the stock, these can include:
- Collard greens
- Eggplant
- Bok choy
- Kale
- Spinach
- Zucchini

Please note that if you're suffering from extreme cases of diarrhea, it is recommended that you exclude vegetables at first and focus on stock with probiotic-rich foods every hour with well-cooked meats and fish. You will not want to introduce vegetables until after the diarrhea begins to calm down. You want to reduce that inflammation before adding in the fiber.

Fermented yogurt & dairy - only include a small amount each day, about one to two teaspoons, and then gradually work your way up to a tablespoon or so after about five days. Only include fermented yogurt if you are not sensitive or allergic to dairy. Homemade is best, and you can find a homemade recipe in the recipe section of this book. You may also want to consider adding in some whey, sour cream, kefir or raw milk (if you do not have a sensitivity to dairy). Again, quality is key here, so you will want to opt for the highest quality possible. This may be a great option for those who suffer from diarrhea.

Other fermented foods - there are other ways to get probiotic-rich foods into your diet. The juice from your homemade sauerkraut or fermented vegetables is an excellent option. Try adding these to your soup for an extra probiotic-rich boost. These are the best fermented options if you suffer from constipation.

Ginger, mint or chamomile tea - you can sweeten your tea with a small amount of raw and local honey if desired. Be sure to use the whole leaf version of tea and not the powdered version.

Once the introduction phase of this diet begins, you can decide to move through the diet as fast as your body permits. You may wish to stay at different stages for different periods of time. For example, you may want to only stay on Stage 1 of the introduction diet for three days but then stay at Stage 2 for 4–5 days. Listen to your body and move through at the pace you feel is best. The most important thing to remember is to take the introduction diet seriously and not to skip it or rush through it. The introduction phase of the GAPS diet is integral to success and, by following this part of the diet, you allow your digestive system to begin the healing process quicker than you would if you completely skipped over it. Stick to each stage of the introduction diet for at least a few days to help improve symptoms before moving to the next stage.

Stage 2

Now that you have made it to Stage 2, you are probably hoping that you can add a bit more into your diet! If you've made it to this stage, you are also probably starting to feel better and you are probably starting to get excited about the amazing possibilities this diet has to heal your gut. If you've had some detoxifying symptoms or "die-off", this is great as well because it is a sign that your body is getting rid of the toxins and getting better. For Stage 2, you will still want to be enjoying your soups boiled with meats, vegetables and probiotic-rich foods. You will probably want to gradually add some raw organic eggs into the soups at this point. It's important to only add the egg yolks into the soups, removing the egg whites. You can start with one egg yolk per day and then gradually increase it until you are enjoying an egg for each bowl of soup you enjoy. Stick with organic, free-range eggs and only include them if you do not have a sensitivity or allergy to eggs. At this stage, you can also add in some stews and casseroles made with meats and vegetables but avoid any spices in Stage 2.

Stage 3

Welcome to Stage 3! You have started adding more foods into your diet, as you steadily increase the amount of probiotic-rich foods in your diet as well. On Stage 3, you will want to continue with the foods you have been eating and you can now add a ripe avocado mashed into your soups. Start with about 1–3 teaspoons per day. You can now even make GAPS-approved pancakes at this stage, made from nut butter, eggs and squash or zucchini! You can find a recipe in the recipes section to get started. You may also start making scrambled eggs, cooked in ghee or pork fat, and served with avocado and even some cooked onion. Lastly, start to actually eat the fermented vegetables and sauerkraut instead of only enjoying the juice. Start small and work your way up to having 1–4 teaspoons at each meal.

Stage 4

At Stage 4, you will want to gradually increase cooked meats by roasting and grilling them instead of only cooking them in your soups. Enjoy cooked meats with cooked vegetables as well as sauerkraut. You can now also begin enjoying freshly-pressed juice by starting with a very small amount of carrot juice. Once you are comfortable having a full cup of fresh carrot juice per day, you can branch out and try celery, cabbage, lettuce and mint juices as well. At Stage 4 you are also welcome to add in cold-pressed olive oil, working your way up to 1–2 tablespoons for each meal. Lastly, you can start to bake with ground almonds by making almond bread or make the bread with any other nuts and seeds ground into flour.

Stage 5

On Stage 5 of the GAPS diet, you will want to continue to enjoy all of the nourishing foods you have already added into your diet and you can begin to add cooked apple puree. Keep an eye out for a recipe in the recipes section! You may also begin adding raw vegetables, starting with the softer parts of lettuce and cucumber. Increase the raw vegetable intake until well tolerated and, if diarrhea comes back, you know your body is not quite ready to introduce these foods yet. If the vegetable juices have been well tolerated, you can now begin to add fruits such as pineapple and mango, but still keep citrus fruits out of your diet at this point.

Stage 6

You have almost completed the GAPS introduction diet! I hope that you are feeling much better and are ready to start the full GAPS diet.

While it may seem like six stages are quite a lot to get through, I hope that breaking down each stage makes things a little clearer. As you can see, each stage builds the stage before it and goes at a gradual pace so as not to trigger any inflammation in your body. As you progress through the diet, remember to keep enjoying the foods from the previous stage as well so you are gradually increasing the variety of food that you are eating. Listen to your body and go at a pace that works for you. Once you have finished all six stages, you are ready for the full GAPS diet, which you will find a breeze by comparison!

Chapter 3: Food to eat and to avoid

The first stages of introduction to the GAPS diet are always harsh. A person needs to work through it slowly in order to change the pathogenic microorganism in your gut. As the microorganisms start vanishing, body reactions will increase which will make you feel unpleasant and want to quit the process. In the process of breaking down and disintegration of the microorganism, toxic substances are going to be released from your body. At the start of the GAPS diet the reactions can get significantly bad but get better later. There are different stages of GAPS diet and, each stage depends on the individual person and how your body adapts to food.

What is usually recommended in stage 1 of GAPS diet is:

- Start by drinking a glass of water in the morning.
- At every meal eat fish stock or meat (fats and soft tissues of the bone marrow).
- Every time you have a meal, drink a glass of natural juice for the fermented food requirement.
- Always eat soup made from stock, that is: leeks, cabbage, greens, pumpkin, squash, broccoli, carrots and other vegetables.
- Tea made from ginger or Mint with a little amount of honey allowed.

- Boiled vegetables, which help in digestion and constipation.
- Coconut oil
- Raw garlic

Once you have entered into stage 2 of the GAPS Diet and your digestion is working smoothly, you can begin to introduce some additional foods into your eating plan.

Remember, you can still eat all of the foods you ate in Phase 1 while working some of these foods into your diet. Raw, organic egg yolks followed by soft boiled eggs are a good place to start. Begin with one organic egg yolk per day and add it to your soup for a bit of extra flavor. Once you know you can tolerate this well, work your way up to soft-boiled eggs.

Stews and casseroles made with meat, vegetables, and animal fat are also a welcome addition to the diet. These will help you to feel full while helping to regulate your system. Although it may be tempting, be sure not to introduce too many spices at this point.

Ghee, or clarified butter, is another delicious addition to this phase of the diet. Ghee can be ordered online, but it is costly so I recommend you make your own. Making Ghee is simple, and there are many recipes online that are easy to follow. I suggest you make a large amount and freeze it. You will save loads of money by doing this and I bet you will never buy butter again!

Being well prepared is key to sticking to this diet. Though the beginning stages may be tough, the benefits will be amazing in the long run.

Protein is very important in the GAPS Diet, with the bones and fat adhered to the meat. Two to three eggs with the yolk still raw every day promotes neurological benefits, and liver and organ meats is highly encouraged because they are extremely nutritious.

All types of fresh or frozen vegetables are included, and they can be steamed, boiled, grilled, roasted or stir-fried. Eating vegetables raw is recommended, but have them separate from the cooked veggies. Fermented vegetables are also encouraged.

Fresh fruit is offered with certain perimeters, and fruit should always be eaten separately because it is digested differently. Avocados are a great with anything, including your choice of meats or salads. They are high in nutrition, a good fat source and simply delicious.

The fifth step of the program allows the patient to consume all of the foods that were tolerated in the first four steps of the program as well as new introduced items.

- Pecan flour
- Apple puree, must be cooked
- Apple juice (use freshly juiced)

- Cucumber, peeled
- Lettuce-soft parts
- Tomatoes, raw only
- Mangoes
- Onions, raw only
- Papaya juice
- Spices-pure, single
- Mango juice
- Walnut flour
- Pineapple juice
- String beans

Remember, you are adding these food items into your GAPS intro diet plan. You have already moved through stages 1, 2, 3 and 4 to get to stage 5. These foods are only to be included once you have completed the other 4 stages of food. You will be able to move onto stage 6 after you have finished with stage 5 with no problems. You may repeat previous stages of the GAPS diet if needed, due to digestive problems.

Though Stage 6 is less restrictive than the previous stages, it still requires some planning. Breakfast can be particularly difficult due to the diet's lack of grains and cereals. Here are a few breakfast ideas to help you out.

Benefits of gaps diet

The purpose of the GAPS diet is to do away with the negative reactions you may be having with food. Over a course consisting of six stages, foods will be reintroduced to your body. The entire course of the GAPS diet normally is six weeks' average. The amount of time the GAPS diet is used is strongly dependent upon the individual's dietary needs.

The GAPS Diet is an amazing way of eating while detoxifying the digestion system. Many people have problems in their gut, and they don't know that there is an answer to the unhealthy and uncomfortable way they are feeling.

The Gut and Psychology Syndrome Diet was developed using the Carbohydrate Diet and adopting new concepts. The diet is often recommended by physicians, and it consists of six stages that will typically take 2.5 years to normalize and return to full foods.

Spring Clean Your Body with the Gaps Diet!

Toxins are everywhere. Most people would like to just take a broom and sweep out all the free radicals, chemicals, and junk that has been accumulating inside their bodies but very few people know how. The Gaps diet incorporates simple steps to ensure your success in ridding your body of harmful fumes and chemicals.

First, get rid of the toxins that are under your control. Sadly, airborne chemicals are a fact of life in the 21st century but you can make your home a haven. Try avoiding new paint or carpet when possible. Another way to cut down on fumes in the air is to rethink your cleaning products. All that bleach, chlorine, and ammonia isn't good for your body. The good news is there are cheap alternatives! Vinegar and baking soda are two cleaning powerhouses that won't produce toxins. Also, consider cleaning the air with living air filter-houseplants!

You've had toxins building up for years. It's time to start adding a few housecleaners for inside your body. The Gaps diet focuses on natural foods that rid your body of free radicals and help scrub the gunk out of your system. Juicing is essential for your success. Get the best of your veggies in its most concentrated form. Your body will thank you.

Living in a toxic world is not always easy, get the Gaps diet on your side and start cleaning from the inside out!

How Does the GAPS Diet Help with IBS?

Irritable Bowel Syndrome is one of the most uncomfortable, inconvenient diseases in existence. In fact, in the United Kingdom, it ranks second in the top reasons employees miss work.

Worse, because the symptoms of IBS can be general and vary in intensity, the disease can be difficult to treat and cure. However, the GAPS diet can do a lot to help people with IBS feel well again and even get rid of their symptoms completely.

The GAPS diet is based around the use of several hard, protein-rich foods and the slow introduction of different food groups over time. For example, it is recommended that patients start with an "introductory diet."

During this phase, he or she is encouraged to start the day with mineral water or vegetable juice and move on to homemade meat or fish broths (stock). On the introductory diet, the patient can also eat joint and bone parts of meat, as well as whole chicken, if prepared according to specifications, and vegetables such as cabbage or celery. All these foods encourage the growth of new stomach cells, which can help repair one's damaged gut lining.

As the person continues with the GAPS diet, he or she can add new foods and food groups, but only as long as the food is tolerable. Doctors who endorse GAPS recommend slowly adding in foods like eggs, particularly egg whites, as well as yogurt, pancakes, and baked goods made with dried fruit.

During the GAPS diet, participants, especially those with IBS, should watch their stools. Ideally, a stool will look like a smooth sausage or snake and glide out with no pushing or straining. Stools that resemble hard nuts indicate the person is eating something harmful or not tolerating some part of the new diet;

stools that are too mushy or are almost entirely liquid indicate the same.

Irritable Bowel Syndrome can be difficult to treat and cure. This is particularly true since many IBS patients have various food sensitivities. Diets like GAPS, however, have been proven to help these patients' symptoms lessen, thus improving their quality of life.

How Does the Gap Diet Affect Constipation, Here's the Truth?

The GAPS diet does not work well for constipation. In some cases, the bowel movement will stop entirely. Dr. Natasha Campbell-McBride says that stopped bowel movement is common in stage 1 of the "Intro Diet."

The start of the GAPS diet has no fiber. None of the stuff that allows bowel movement. Apparently, for some people, fiber is actually the source of the problem. Fiber cleans out your system, but for some, it is a real irritant. Success rates vary depending on the source you attain them from. Either way, you look at it, it all depends on your own health condition.

By going out on your faith that this theory works, you genuinely believe that it is doing healing work. There are always positives and negatives to any diet. The diet may heal and fix some constipation, but not many. Balance the good and the bad with a doctor and see if it can really help, but someone should never go out on a limb without evidence.

This is, however, a rare case. Most people need more fiber, not less. Some people only eat meat, so of course, these diets wouldn't do much good for those people. So this diet only relieves constipation on a select few people. Using an enema is a choice, but why would anyone pay for something they don't have to? Recommendation is to consult a doctor and figure out what the problem. Then, if it is caused by fiber irritant, then go ahead. If not, take actions to fix the problem.

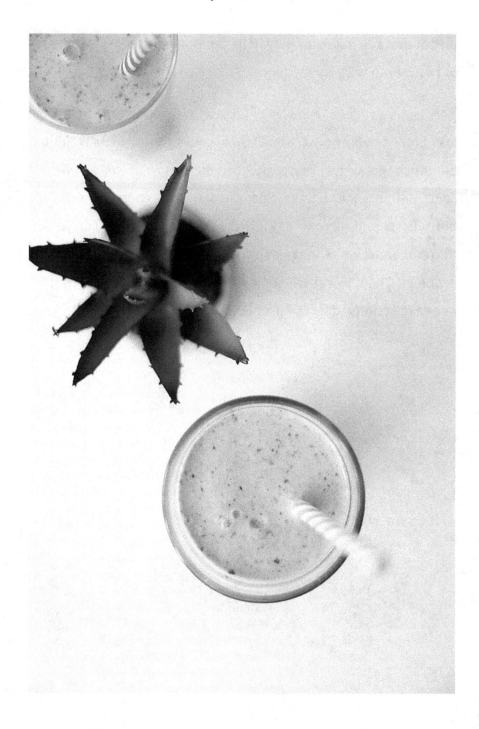

Chapter 4: supplementation

Most of the time, your body can't do healing on its own. This is particularly true in cases where damage has been extensive or your gut isn't strong enough to recover by itself. This makes supplementation necessary.

Deglycyrrhizinated Licorice

Licorice root has been a part of traditional medicine for several years already. It has both anti-inflammatory and antibacterial property. However, with prolonged use, licorice has been closely linked with cases of hypertension and other adverse reactions.

Deglycyrrhizinated licorice, or DGL, is created out of whole licorice but underwent further processing to remove Glycyrrhizin which largely contributes to elevated blood pressure. DGL, as a supplement, supports the proliferation of the mucus secreting cells of the gut and prolong gastric cellular life. It also improves the circulation in the gut and assist in its healing. DGL is effective to use in cases of peptic ulcers as well as Gastro-intestinal Reflux Disease.

Betaine Hydrochloric Acid

Low levels of stomach acid can lead to several problems. Primarily, an acidic environment is needed to make sure bad bacteria don't proliferate. Indigestion, acid reflux and nutrient deficiencies are also caused by insufficient acid in the stomach.

To compensate for this, you can supplement with Betaine Hydrochloric Acid. This supplement helps increase the acidity and amount of acid in your stomach. Although helpful with people who don't produce enough HCL in their gut, there are also people who need to skip this supplement. This includes people who are under corticosteroid therapy and those suffering from ulcers of the digestive track.

L-Glutamine

L-Glutamine is essentially a form of amino acid. It helps the body synthesize nucleic acid as well as protein. In terms of your gut health, L-Glutamine works to protect the mucosal lining of your digestive track. It also decreases the proliferation of bad bacteria while preventing natural cell death in the area.

Because of these properties, L-Glutamine is considered as effective in managing or even reversing the damages created by the leaky gut syndrome. Because the condition primarily affects the lining of the gut and its ability to serve as a barrier, you can rely on glutamine as support.

Slippery Elm

Slippery elm comes from the inner bark of the elm tree. It's widely used in parts of Northern America to relieve ailments, particularly of the digestive track. Slippery elm triggers natural mucus secretion. Mucus, as we all know, is important in that it coats and protects the lining of the gut. This mechanism helps greatly in avoiding ulcer formation as well as in preventing further damage to existing ulcers.

This supplement also aids in removing toxins inside your gut. It helps hasten food processing and the time it takes to transfer the food in the track. Aside from this, slippery elm also has the ability to add bulk and soften stool to facilitate easier elimination. It's equally effective in reducing inflammation and irritation in the gut caused by Irritable Bowel Syndrome and colitis.

Digestive Enzymes

Digestive enzymes naturally occur in your gut to help break down food into a form that it can easily absorb. If these enzymes become insufficient, such as with age or certain diseases, the gastrointestinal track becomes less efficient with its job. Not all digestive enzyme supplements are created equal. If you are new to purchasing this type of supplement, you should be looking out for one that has enzymes capable of helping you digest protein, fats and carbohydrates.

Aloe Vera

Aloe Vera is good for your skin. It's an effective moisturizer and a scar remover. Aside from these benefits, aloe Vera is also good for your digestive health. Primarily, it helps enhance digestion through its cleansing effect on the gut. This effect is not only limited to your stomach or your duodenum but the entire digestive track. Aloe Vera has an anti-inflammatory effect and can soothe ulcers and irritated gastric linings. If you are suffering from constipation, taking aloe Vera can help you as it is also considered an effective laxative.

Aloe Vera can be used fresh. It's actually the safer means of reaping the benefits of the plant. However, if you don't have immediate access to aloe Vera plant, you always have the option to buy from suppliers. If you are taking it in supplement form, take time and exercise caution in studying the brand and the supplement. You should also be aware of how much and how long you're allowed to take aloe Vera supplements. Most of the time, your attending health care specialist can give you an exact duration.

Chapter 5: Breakfast Recipe

1. Mango Green Tea Shake

Preparation Time: 5 minutes

Cooking Time: 5 minutes

Servings: 1

Ingredients:

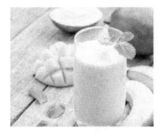

1 cup mango, cubed

1 teaspoon fresh grated ginger

1 tablespoon honey

½ cup fresh brewed green tea

1 cup coconut yogurt 1 cup ice

Directions:

Place all of the ingredients in a blender.

Blend until smooth and creamy.

Enjoy immediately in a chilled glass.

Nutrition: Calories: 61 Protein: 4 G Fat: 3 G Carbs: 6 G

2. Minty Papaya Smoothie

Preparation Time: 5 minutes

Cooking Time: 5 minutes

Servings: 1

Ingredients:

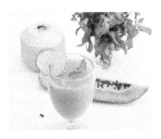

1 cup papaya, cubed

1 banana, cubed

1 teaspoon lime juice

1 teaspoon fresh mint

1 cup dairy kefir

1 cup ice

Directions:

Place all of the ingredients in a blender.

Blend until smooth and creamy.

Enjoy immediately in a chilled glass.

Nutrition: Calories 169, Fat 6.5 g, Fiber 2.6 g, Carbs 10.6 g, Protein 9.4 g

3. Cocoa Banana Protein Power

Preparation Time: 5 minutes

Cooking Time: 5 minutes

Servings: 1

Ingredients:

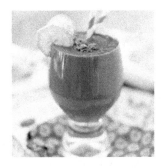

1 medium banana, cubed

1 tablespoon almond butter

½ teaspoon cinnamon

1 tablespoon chocolate protein powder

1 cup dairy kefir

1 cup ice

Directions:

Place all of the ingredients in a blender.

Blend until smooth and creamy.

Enjoy immediately in a chilled glass.

4. Slow-cooked Peppers Frittata

Preparation Time: 10 minutes

Cooking Time: 3 hours

Servings: 6

Ingredients:

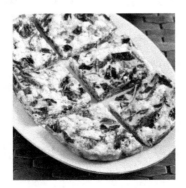

½ cup almond milk

8 eggs, whisked

Salt and black pepper to the taste

1 teaspoon oregano, dried

1 and ½ cups roasted peppers, chopped

½ cup red onion, chopped

4 cups baby arugula

1 cup goat cheese, crumbled

Cooking spray

Directions:

In a bowl, combine the eggs with salt, pepper, and the oregano and whisk.

Grease your slow cooker with the cooking spray, arrange the peppers and the remaining ingredients inside and pour the egg mixture over them.

Put the lid on and cook on Low for 3 hours.

Divide the frittata between plates and serve.

Nutrition: Calories: 259 Protein: 16 G Fat: 20 G Carbs: 4.4 G

5. Veggie Bowls

Preparation Time: 10 minutes

Cooking Time: 5 minutes

Servings: 4

Ingredients:

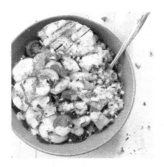

tablespoon olive oil

1 pound asparagus, trimmed and roughly chopped

3 cups kale, shredded

3 cups Brussels sprouts, shredded

½ cup hummus

1 avocado, peeled, pitted and sliced

4 eggs, soft boiled, peeled and sliced

2 tablespoons lemon juice

1 garlic clove, minced

2 teaspoons Dijon mustard

2 tablespoons olive oil

Salt and black pepper to the taste

Directions:

Heat up a pan with 2 tablespoons oil over medium-high heat, add the asparagus and sauté for 5 minutes stirring often.

In a bowl, combine the other 2 tablespoons oil with the lemon juice, garlic, mustard, salt, and pepper and whisk well.

In a salad bowl, combine the asparagus with the kale, sprouts, hummus, avocado, and the eggs and toss gently.

Add the dressing, toss, and serve for breakfast.

Nutrition: Calories: 323 Protein: 27 G Fat: 21 G Carbs: 25 G

6. Simple Steel Cuts

Preparation Time: 5 minutes

Cooking Time: 10 minutes

Servings: 4

Ingredients:

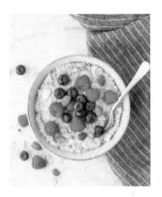

½ cup steel cut oats

2 cups of water

1 tablespoon oil

Dash of salt

Directions:

Add the listed ingredients to the Instant Pot.

up the lid and cook on HIGH pressure for 10 minutes.

Lock Release the pressure naturally. Top it up with granola, dried fruit or nuts. Enjoy! Add a bit of maple syrup or agave syrup for sweetness

Nutrition: Calories 200 Fat 7.6 Fiber 2.5 Carbs 5.5 Protein 4.5

7. Vanilla Flavored Oats

Preparation Time: 10 minutes

Cooking Time: 10 minutes

Servings: 4

Ingredients:

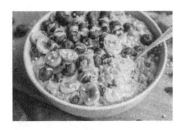

1 cup almond milk

2 and ½ cups of water

1 cup old fashioned oats

2 tablespoons coconut sugar

1 teaspoon espresso powder

2 teaspoons vanilla extract

Directions:

Vanilla flavored oats are the ones to go for! Add milk, oats, sugar, espresso, vanilla extract to your Instant Pot and toss.

Close lid and cook on HIGH pressure for 10 minutes.

Release pressure naturally over 10 minutes.

Stir and divide into serving bowls.

Serve and enjoy!

Nutrition: Calories 192 Fat 3.4 Fiber 4.5 Carbs 7.6 Protein 3.5

8. Feta Baked Eggs

Preparation Time: 5 minutes

Cooking Time: 10 minutes

Servings: 4

Ingredients:

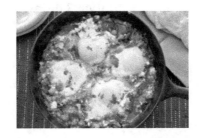

4 whole eggs

4 slices feta

2 spring onions, chopped

1 cup of water

1 tablespoon olive oil

1 tablespoon cilantro, chopped

Directions:

The original breakfast dish, simple feta dressed baked eggs!
Grease 4 ramekins with oil and sprinkle green onion in each.

Crack an egg into each and top with cilantro and cheese.

Add water to your Pot. Place a steamer basket. Place ramekin inside and cover.

Cook on LOW pressure for 4 minutes. Release pressure naturally.

Serve and enjoy!

Nutrition: Calories 193 Fat 5.4 Fiber 3.4 Carbs 7.6 Protein 3

9. Buckwheat Porridge

Preparation Time: 5 minutes

Cooking Time: 6 minutes

Servings: 4

Ingredients:

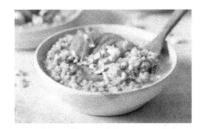

½ cup raisins

3 cups of rice milk

1 banana, peeled and sliced

½ teaspoon vanilla extract

1 cup buckwheat groats, rinsed

Directions:

Everybody goes for oats but why should you do the same? Try a delicious Buckwheat porridge for a change! Add buckwheat to your Pot.

Add raisins, milk, banana, vanilla and stir.

Close lid and cook on HIGH pressure for 6 minutes.

Release the pressure naturally over 10 minutes.

Enjoy!

Nutrition: Calories 122 Fat 5.7 Fiber 3.2 Carbs 5.3 Protein 0.4

Chapter 6: Snack Recipes

10. Creamy Butternut Porridge

Preparation Time: 10 minutes

Cooking Time: 25 minutes

Servings: 3

Ingredients:

2 cups butternut squash, peeled and cubed

4 tbsp coconut kefir

1/4 tsp sea salt

Directions:

Cook butternut squash in water until tender.

Add cooked butternut squash, salt and kefir in blender and blend until creamy.

Serve and enjoy.

Nutrition: calories 270, fat 18g, fiber 1g, carbs 3g, protein 22g

11.　　Avocado and Sauerkraut

Preparation Time: 5 minutes

Cooking Time: 0 minutes

Servings: 1

Ingredients:

¼ avocado, pitted and mashed

1 tsp. homemade sauerkraut

1 pinch of Celtic sea salt

Directions:

Slice the avocado and mash with the sauerkraut.

Season with salt and enjoy right away.

Tip:The recipe for homemade sauerkraut can be found in the base recipes section.

Nutrition: calories 298, fat 12g, fiber 2g, carbs 20g, protein 5g

12.   Onion Egg Scramble

Preparation Time: 10 minutes

Cooking Time: 20 minutes

Servings: 4

Ingredients:

4 organic pasture-raised eggs, whisked

¼ cup white onion, chopped

4 Tbsp. grass-fed ghee

Pinch of Celtic sea salt

Directions:

Start by heating the ghee in a pan over low heat and add the onion. Cover the pan and cook for about 20 minutes.

Add the eggs and scramble until cooked. Mix the onions in well whilst stirring.

Serve with a pinch of salt and enjoy.

Nutrition: calories 298, fat 12g, fiber 2g, carbs 20g, protein 5g

13.   Lacto-Fermented Carrots

Preparation Time: 10 minutes

Cooking Time: 0 minutes

Servings: 12

Ingredients:

2 cups filtered water

2 lb. carrots, sliced

1½ Tbsp. Celtic sea salt

2 Tbsp. fresh dill, chopped

Directions:

Start by dissolving the salt in the 2 cups of water in a large mixing bowl.

Add the carrots to a mason style glass jar and fill with the water.

Add the fresh dill to the jar.

Cover the jar and allow it to sit for 2 days. After two days, carefully release some of the air from the jar by unscrewing the cap and letting just a small amount of air out. This is called "burping"

Allow the carrots to ferment for about 7 days, "burping" the jars every couple of days.

Store the carrots in the refrigerator and enjoy as an easy on-the-go snack.

Nutrition: calories 270, fat 18g, fiber 1g, carbs 3g, protein 22g

14.   Almond Cake

Preparation Time: 20 minutes

Cooking Time: 60 minutes

Servings: 10

Ingredients:

250 g softened dairy free butter

75 g castor sugar

4 eggs

240 g finely ground almonds

40 g rice flour

Low FODMAP cream to serve

Direction:

Preheat the oven to 320° F

Grease a pan, 6 cm deep and 22 cm round and then line it with baking paper

Beat the butter and the sugar using a hand mixer, until light and fluffy

Add the eggs one at a time, beating after each one

Stir the finely chopped almonds and flour into the mix

Spread over the pan and bake for 75 minutes or until cooked through

Leave to cool in the pan for 10 minutes, then turn out onto a wire rack and cool for a further 10 minute

Serves with the cream and fresh fruit of your choice

Nutrition: calories 200, fat 8g, fiber 4g, carbs 8g, protein 3g

15.　　Instant Banana Pudding

Preparation time: 10 minutes

Cooking time: 10 minutes

Serves 12

Ingredients:

140 g box of Jell-O vanilla instant pudding

600 ml lactose free milk

150 g pack of gluten free cookies

3 whole bananas, peeled

Direction:

Whisk the pudding mix and milk together for 2 minutes until the pudding begins to thicken

Place in the refrigerator to continue thickening

Slice the bananas and divide into two piles

Break up the cookies and spread half of them over the base of an 8 x 8 pan

Place half of the bananas over the top and follow with half of the pudding mix

Repeat with the rest of the ingredients

Nutrition: calories 110, fat 10g, fiber 1g, carbs 3g, protein 6g

16.   Chocolate-Orange-Raspberry Cupcakes

Preparation time: 15 minutes

Cooking time: 30 minutes

Serving : 12

Ingredients:

360 ml almond milk

120 ml unsweetened orange juice

1 tsp rice vinegar

450 g Turbinado sugar

160 ml vegetable oil

2 eggs

200 g oat flour

½ tsp xanthan gum

35 g cocoa powder

1 tsp baking soda

1 tsp baking powder

½ tsp salt

2 tsp orange zest

2 tbsp. organic raspberry preserves

1 tsp vanilla

Direction:

Preheat oven to 350° F

Line a cupcake tin with molds

Mix the vinegar, milk and orange juice together and leave to curdle for 5 minutes

Mic the flour, xanthan gum, baking powder, baking soda, cocoa and salt together

Beat the eggs in a separate bowl with the oil, sugar and orange zest

Mix the flour mix and the milk into the egg mix, alternating each one to ensure even mixing and beat until the mixture is smooth and well combined

Spoon into the molds and bake for 30 minutes

Leave to cool while you make the frosting

Nutrition: calories 383, fat 14g, fiber 4g, carbs 3g, protein 8g

17.   Chocolate-Orange-Raspberry Frosting

Preparation Time: 10 minutes

Cooking Time: 10 minutes

Servings: 4

Ingredients:

770 g sifted powdered sugar

2 tbsp. unsweetened cocoa powder

½ tsp salt

60 ml almond milk

675 g dairy-free butter

1 tsp vanilla extract

1 tbsp. orange juice

2 tsp organic raspberry preserves

Orange zest - for flavor and/or garnish

Direction:

Mix the sugar with the salt and cocoa powder

Using an electric mixer, mix the milk, orange juice and raspberry jelly together for about 5 minutes or until smooth

Add the vanilla and butter and beat for a further 10 minutes

Frost the cupcakes and serve

Nutrition: calories 333, fat 1g, fiber 1g, carbs 6g, protein 2g

18.   Graham Crackers

Preparation time: 140 minutes

Cooking time: 20 minutes

Serving : 3

Ingredients:

325 g all purpose flour, gluten free, sifted

2 extra tbsp. gluten free all-purpose flour

2 ½ tsp xanthan gum

170 g dark brown sugar

1 tsp baking soda

¾ tsp coarse sea salt

7 tbsp. dairy free butter – cut into cubes of 1" and freeze in advance

90 g molasses

5 tablespoons lactose free whole milk

2 tbsp. clear vanilla extract

3 tbsp. granulated sugar

1 tsp ground cinnamon

Direction:

Mix the flour together with the xanthan gum, brown sugar, baking soda, and salt in a food processor using a steel blade or in and electric mixer using the paddle

Either pule or lave on a low setting to thoroughly mix

Ass in the frozen cubes of butter and pulse until the mixture looks like coarse meal

Whisk the vanilla, molasses and milk together in a separate bowl

Add the liquid into the dry mixture and pulse until the mixture is a soft and sticky dough that only just comes together

Dust a large piece of plastic wrap with flour (gluten free) and turn the dough out onto it

Pat and shape into a 1" thick rectangle, wrap it up and chill in the refrigerator until firm, around 2 hours

Mix the granulated sugar and the cinnamon together and leave to one side

When the dough is chilled divide it in half and put half back in the refrigerator

Sprinkle flour evenly on the work surface and roll out the dough into a long rectangle, around 1/8" thick. It will be sticky so use more flour as and when you need it but make sure it is gluten freeCut the dough up into rectangles that are 4 ½" by 4" approximately

Place them onto a baking sheet lined with baking paper and sprinkle the sugar and cinnamon mix over the top ad place in the refrigerator for about 30-45 minutes or until firm (alternatively, pop the tray in the freezer for 15-20 minutes)

Repeat the process with the other half of the dough and then, with any scraps that are left over

While the crackers are chilling, preheat the oven to 350° F

Bake the crackers for 15-25 minutes or until they have browned and are a little firm to the touch. Make sure you rotate the baking trays halfway through cooking to make sure they are evenly baked

Nutrition: calories 200, fat 8g, fiber 4g, carbs 8g, protein 3g

Chapter 7: Lunch recipes

19.   Avocado Salmon Salad

Preparation Time: 10 minutes

Cooking Time: 0 minutes

Servings: 4

Ingredients:

2 ripe avocados, mashed

2 (3 ounce) wild caught salmon filets, cooked, and flaked

1 large carrot, peeled and shredded

2 cups spinach, finely chopped

2 Tbsp. lemon juice

½ tsp. mineral salt

Directions:

In a large bowl, add the avocado and mash with a fork. Add the remaining ingredients and mix to combine.

Serve on a slice of GAPS bread or on top of greens.

Nutrition: calories 283, fat 8g, fiber 1g, carbs 3g, protein 9g

20.   Chicken Taco Salad

Preparation Time: 15 minutes

Cooking Time: 0 minutes

Servings: 4

Ingredients:

¼ cup cold-pressed olive oil

2 Tbsp. lime juice

1 tsp. mineral salt

1 tsp. garlic powder

1 tsp. ground cumin

½ tsp. onion powder

½ tsp. paprika

¼ tsp. oregano

1 lb. chicken, cooked and shredded

4 cups romaine lettuce, chopped

1 tomato, chopped

1 red bell pepper, chopped

½ cup cilantro, chopped

1 avocado, sliced

Directions:

In a large bowl, whisk together the olive oil, lime juice, salt and spices.

Add the remaining ingredients and toss to combine.

Serve topped with sliced avocado.

Nutrition: calories 555, fat 28g, fiber 2g, carbs 6g, protein 27g

21.   African Chicken Peanut Stew

Preparation Time: 10 minutes

Cooking Time: 40 minutes

Servings: 6

Ingredients:

2 Tbsp. homemade ghee

1 onion, chopped

1 tsp. mineral salt

1 red bell pepper, chopped

2 cups butternut squash, peeled and cut into bite-sized cubes

2 cloves garlic

1 tsp. ground turmeric

1 Tbsp. fresh ginger, minced

½ tsp. ground coriander

½ tsp. ground cinnamon

2 cups homemade tomato purée

2 cups homemade coconut milk

1 cup homemade meat stock

1 ½ lb. chicken thighs, boneless and skinless

½ cup peanut butter

2 cups kale, chopped

Fresh cilantro (for topping)

Chopped peanuts (for topping)

Lime wedges (for topping)

Directions:

In a large skillet, melt the ghee over a medium heat. Add the onion and salt and cook until softened, for about 5 minutes. Add the red bell pepper, butternut squash, garlic, turmeric, ginger, coriander and cinnamon. Cook for 30 seconds, stirring constantly.

Add the tomato purée, coconut milk, stock and chicken. Simmer, uncovered, for 30 minutes, or until the chicken is cooked through.

Transfer the chicken to a cutting board and shred the meat, then return to the pot. Stir in the peanut butter and kale and simmer for an additional 2 minutes.

Serve topped with cilantro, peanuts and a lime wedge.

Nutrition: calories 283, fat 8g, fiber 1g, carbs 3g, protein 9g

22.　　**Hawaiian Toastie**

Preparation Time: 10 minutes

Cooking Time: 6 minutes

Servings: 1

Ingredients:

2 slices spelt sourdough or wheat bread

35 grams cheddar cheese, grated

2 tablespoons green onions

2 tablespoons butter

30 grams shaved ham, sliced

40 grams canned pineapple chunks, rinsed and drained

Black pepper

Directions

Chop the pineapple chunks.

Remove the white stem of the green onions and chop the green tips finely.

Spread butter on one side of both bread slices. Place cheese, pineapple, ham and green onions on top of the buttered side of the bread. Season with black pepper to taste.

Place the other bread slice on top to completely assemble the toastie.

Heat the toastie for about 3 minutes or until it becomes golden brown in color.

Nutrition: calories 323, fat 11g, fiber 4g, carbs 13g, protein 17g

23.   Chicken Alfredo Pasta Bake

Preparation Time: 10 minutes

Cooking Time: 50 minutes

Servings: 4

Ingredients:

450 grams chicken breast

3 tablespoons fresh sage, chopped

5 tablespoons butter

114 grams cheddar cheese, grated

¼ cup plain flour, gluten-free

20 grams green onions

750 milliliters rice milk

180 grams broccoli florets

3 tablespoons parmesan cheese, grated

120 grams baby spinach, chopped

½ teaspoon basil, dried

240 grams pasta, gluten-free

Salt and pepper

Olive oil

Directions

Heat the oven to 180 degrees Celsius. Apply olive oil on a large oven dish to grease it.

Slice the chicken breast fillet into small pieces. Sear the chicken using olive oil in a large frying pan over medium-high heat. Once the meat is golden brown, remove it from the flame and set aside for later.

Remove the white stems of the green onions and chop the green tips finely.

Place the spinach leaves in a hot pan until slightly wilted. Remove from heat and place it on one side for later use.

Over medium heat, melt the butter in a medium-sized saucepan. Add plain flour into the saucepan and stir continuously for a minute while cooking.

Once slightly frothy, add ½ cup of milk into the saucepan and stir until smooth. Pour 1 cup of milk at a time into the mixture while stirring continuously. Season to taste.

Add parmesan cheese, basil and 57 grams of cheddar cheese into the sauce. Give the mixture an occasional stir until it gained a thick consistency.

Prepare a large saucepan of boiling water and cook the pasta.

After 5 minutes, drain the pasta and drizzle with olive oil. Add Alfredo sauce, broccoli, chicken and spinach into the pasta and mix well.

Transfer everything to the greased oven dish and sprinkle the remaining cheese on top.

Let it cook in the oven for 10 minutes without cover. Place the pasta bake in an oven grill and cook for another 3 minutes. Garnish with sage.

Nutrition: calories 754, fat 14g, fiber 2g, carbs 16g, protein 26g

24.   Lamb Deal

Preparation Time: 15 minutes

Cooking Time: 40 minutes

Servings:5

Ingredients:

1 large Onion, cut into wedges

1 large Zucchini, peeled, seeded and cut into wedges

1 large Yellow Squash, seeded and cut into wedges

1 Red Bell Pepper, seeded and cut into chunks

1 Green Bell Pepper, seeded and cut into chunks

1 Orange Bell Pepper, seeded and cut into chunks

Natural unprocessed Salt, to taste

Freshly Crushed Black Pepper, to taste

1 tablespoon Ghee, melted

8 Organic Lean Lamb Chops

2 tablespoons finely diced fresh Rosemary Leaves

1 tablespoon finely diced fresh Thyme Leaves

Directions:

Preheat the oven to 425 degrees F and line a roasting pan. Place the onion, zucchini, squash and bell peppers in the prepared roasting pan. Sprinkle with black pepper and salt, and drizzle with the melted ghee. Roast for 20 minutes.

Meanwhile, in a bowl mix together the salt, black pepper, rosemary and thyme. Add the chops and generously coat with mixture.

Remove the roasting pan from the oven. Push the vegetables to the side and add the chops to the pan. Bake for 20 minutes, turning the chops after 10 minutes.

Serve the chops with the vegetables.

Nutrition: calories 210g, fat 12g, fiber 2g, carbs 8g, protein 6g

25. Baked Beef Casserole

Preparation Time: 5 minutes

Cooking Time: 6 hours

Servings:5

Ingredients:

1 pound Organic Beef Stew Meat

3 large Carrots, peeled and cut into chunks

2 cups Tomatoes, chopped

1 medium Onion, chopped

1 stalk Celery, chopped

¼ teaspoon fresh Rosemary, minced

¼ teaspoon fresh Marjoram, minced

¼ teaspoon fresh Thyme, minced

Natural unprocessed Salt, to taste

Freshly Crushed Black Pepper, to taste ¼ cup Red Wine

Directions:

Preheat the oven to 250 degrees F.

In a casserole dish, place all of the ingredients and mix well.

Cover and bake for 5 to 6 hours, occasionally stirring.

Nutrition: calories 191, fat 9g, fiber 2g, carbs 8g, protein 20g

26.   **Carrot Baked Chicken**

Preparation Time: 15 minutes

Cooking Time: 40 minutes

Servings:5

Ingredients:

1 large Onion, cut into bite size pieces

1 stalk Celery, cut into bite size pieces

3 Carrots, peeled and cut into bite size pieces

1 cup small Broccoli Florets 1 tablespoon White Vinegar

2 tablespoons Extra Virgin Olive Oil

Natural unprocessed Salt, to taste

Freshly Crushed Black Pepper, to taste

½ teaspoon Dried Thyme, crushed

½ teaspoon Dried Oregano, crushed 1 pound Organic Chicken Thighs

Directions:

Preheat the oven to 425 degrees F and lightly grease a baking dish.

Place all of the vegetables in the prepared pan. Drizzle with vinegar and half of the oil. Sprinkle with salt, black pepper and herbs.

Brush the chicken with the remaining oil, and sprinkle with black pepper and salt. Arrange the chicken thighs over the vegetables and bake for 1 hour. Transfer the chicken onto a plate and cover with foil to keep warm.

Mix together the vegetables and bake for a further 5 to 10 minutes. Serve the chicken with the vegetables.

Nutrition: calories 210, fat 8g, fiber 2g, carbs 8g, protein 7g

Chapter 8: Dinner Recipes

27.   Baked Lemon-Butter Fish

Preparation Time: 10 minutes

Cooking Time: 20 minutes

Servings: 2

Ingredients:

4 tablespoons butter, plus more for coating

2 (5-ounce) tilapia fillets

Pink Himalayan salt

Freshly ground black pepper

2 garlic cloves, minced

1 lemon, zested and juiced

2 tablespoons capers, rinsed and chopped

Directions:

Preheat the oven to 400°F. Coat an 8-inch baking dish with butter. Pat dry the tilapia with paper towels, and season on both sides with pink Himalayan salt and pepper. Place in the prepared baking dish. In a medium skillet over medium heat, melt the butter. Add the garlic and cook for 3 to 5 minutes, until slightly browned but not burned. Remove the garlic butter from the heat, and mix in the lemon zest and 2 tablespoons of lemon juice. Pour the lemon-butter sauce over the fish, and sprinkle the capers around the baking pan. Bake for 12 to 15 minutes, until the fish is just cooked through, and serve.

Tip :You could use any mild white fish with this recipe. Even salmon is delicious with the lemon-butter sauce.

Nutrition: calories 103g, fat 4g, fiber 1g, carbs 3g, protein 22g

28.   Fish Taco Bowl

Preparation Time: 10 minutes

Cooking Time: 15 minutes

Servings: 2

Ingredients:

2 (5-ounce) tilapia fillets

1 tablespoon olive oil

2 cups presliced coleslaw cabbage mix

1 avocado, mashed

Pink Himalayan salt

Freshly ground black pepper

4 teaspoons Tajín seasoning salt, divided

1 tablespoon Spicy Red Pepper Miso Mayo, plus more for serving

Directions:

This Fish Taco Bowl makes the most of just a few ingredients, with exciting punches of chile, lime, and red pepper from the Tajín seasoning salt.

The coleslaw mix is a time-saver, and I absolutely love the crunch of the cabbage mixed with the smooth avocado. Preheat the oven to 425°F. Line a baking sheet with aluminum foil or a silicone baking mat. Rub the tilapia with the olive oil, and then coat it with 2 teaspoons of Tajín seasoning salt.

Place the fish in the prepared pan. Bake for 15 minutes, or until the fish is opaque when you pierce it with a fork. Put the fish on a cooling rack and let it sit for 4 minutes.

Meanwhile, in a medium bowl, gently mix to combine the coleslaw and the mayo sauce. You don't want the cabbage super wet, just enough to dress it.

Add the mashed avocado and the remaining 2 teaspoons of Tajín seasoning salt to the coleslaw, and season with pink Himalayan salt and pepper.

Divide the salad between two bowls. Use two forks to shred the fish into small pieces, and add it to the bowls. Top the fish with a drizzle of mayo sauce and serve.

Nutrition: calories 103g, fat 4g, fiber 1g, carbs 3g, protein 22g

29. Scallops With Creamy Bacon Sauce

Preparation Time: 5 minutes

Cooking Time: 20 minutes

Servings: 2

Ingredients:

4 bacon slices

1 cup heavy (whipping) cream

1 tablespoon butter

¼ cup grated Parmesan cheese

Pink Himalayan salt

Freshly ground black pepper

1 tablespoon ghee

8 large sea scallops, rinsed and patted dry

Directions:

When looking for them, choose sea scallops, which are much larger than bay scallops, and avoid frozen scallops, which are harder to work with. Don't forget to remove the small side muscle from the sea scallops before rinsing.

In a medium skillet over medium-high heat, cook the bacon on both sides until crispy, about 8 minutes. Transfer the bacon to a paper towel–lined plate. Lower the heat to medium.

Add the cream, butter, and Parmesan cheese to the bacon grease, and season with a pinch of pink Himalayan salt and pepper. Reduce the heat to low and cook, stirring constantly, until the sauce thickens and is reduced by 50 percent, about 10 minutes.

In a separate large skillet over medium-high heat, heat the ghee until sizzling. Season the scallops with pink Himalayan salt and pepper, and add them to the skillet. Cook for just 1 minute per side.

Do not crowd the scallops; if your pan isn't large enough, cook them in two batches. You want the scallops golden on each side. Transfer the scallops to a paper towel–lined plate.

Divide the cream sauce between two plates, crumble the bacon on top of the cream sauce, and top with 4 scallops each. Serve immediately.

Nutrition: calories 110, fat 10g, fiber 1g, carbs 3g, protein 6g

30.   Beef stew

Preparation Time: 15 minutes

Cooking Time: 60 minutes

Servings: 4

Ingredients

2 lb. beef

1 tsp salt

4 tablespoons olive oil

2 red onions

2 cloves garlic

1 cup white wine

2 cups beef broth

1 cup water

3-4 bay leaves

¼ tsp thyme 1 lb. potatoes

Directions

Chop all ingredients in big chunks

In a large pot heat olive oil and add ingredients one by one

Cook for 5-6 or until slightly brown

Add remaining ingredients and cook until tender, 35-45 minutes

Season while stirring on low heat

When ready remove from heat and serve

Nutrition: calories 280, fat 8g, fiber 3g, carbs 8g, protein 6g

31.   Irish stew

Preparation Time: 10 minutes

Cooking Time: 40 minutes

Servings: 4

Ingredients

4-5 slices bacon

2 lb. beef

¼ cup flour

½ tsp black pepper

4 carrots

½ cup beef broth

Directions

Chop all ingredients in big chunks

In a large pot heat olive oil and add ingredients one by one

Cook for 5-6 or until slightly brown

Add remaining ingredients and cook until tender, 35-45 minutes

Season while stirring on low heat

When ready remove from heat and serve

Nutrition: calories 280, fat 8g, fiber 3g, carbs 8g, protein 6g

32.   Linguine and Brussels sprouts

Preparation time: 10 minutes

Cooking time: 25 minute

Servings: 4

Ingredients:

8 ounces whole-wheat linguine

⅓ cup, plus 2 tablespoons extra-virgin olive oil, divided

1 medium sweet onion, diced

2 to 3 garlic cloves, smashed

8 ounces Brussels sprouts, chopped

½ cup chicken stock, as needed

⅓ cup dry white wine

½ cup shredded Parmesan cheese

1 lemon, cut in quarters

Direction:

Bring a large pot of water to a boil and cook the pasta according to package directions. Drain, reserving 1 cup of the pasta water.

Mix the cooked pasta with 2 tablespoons of olive oil, then set aside.

In a large sauté pan or skillet, heat the remaining ⅓ cup of olive oil on medium heat. Add the onion to the pan and cook for about 5 minutes, until softened. Add the smashed garlic cloves and cook for 1 minute, until fragrant.

Add the Brussels sprouts and cook covered for 15 minutes. Add chicken stock as needed to prevent burning. Once Brussels sprouts have wilted and are fork-tender, add white wine and cook down for about 7 minutes, until reduced.

Add the pasta to the skillet and add the pasta water as needed.

Serve with the Parmesan cheese and lemon for squeezing over the dish right before eating.

Nutrition: Calories: 530; Carbs: 95.4g; Protein: 5.0g; Fat: 16.5g

33. Rustic Vegetable and Brown Rice Bowl

Preparation time: 15 minutes

Cooking time: 10 minute

Servings: 4

Ingredients:

Nonstick cooking spray

2 cups broccoli florets

2 cups cauliflower florets

1 (15-ounce) can chickpeas, drained and rinsed

1 cup carrots sliced 1 inch thick

2 to 3 tablespoons extra-virgin olive oil, divided

Salt

Freshly ground black pepper

2 to 3 tablespoons sesame seeds, for garnish

2 cups cooked brown rice

For the dressing

3 to 4 tablespoons tahini

2 tablespoons honey

1 lemon, juiced

1 garlic clove, minced

Salt

Freshly ground black pepper

Direction:

Preheat the oven to 400°F. Spray two baking sheets with cooking spray.

Cover the first baking sheet with the broccoli and cauliflower and the second with the chickpeas and carrots. Toss each sheet with half of the oil and season with salt and pepper before placing in oven.

Cook the carrots and chickpeas for 10 minutes, leaving the carrots still just crisp, and the broccoli and cauliflower for 20 minutes, until tender. Stir each halfway through cooking.

To make the dressing, in a small bowl, mix the tahini, honey, lemon juice, and garlic. Season with salt and pepper and set aside.

Divide the rice into individual bowls, then layer with vegetables and drizzle dressing over the dish.

Nutrition: Calories: 192; Carbs: 12.7g; Protein: 3.8g; Fat: 15.5g

34.   **Roasted Brussels sprouts And Pecans**

Preparation time: 10 minutes

Cooking time: 15 minute

Servings: 4

Ingredients:

1 ½ pounds fresh Brussels sprouts

4 tablespoons olive oil

4 cloves of garlic, minced

3 tablespoons water

Salt and pepper to taste

½ cup chopped pecans

Directions:

Place all ingredients in the Instant Pot.

Combine all ingredients until well combined.

Close the lid and make sure that the steam release vent is set to "Venting."

Press the "Slow Cook" button and adjust the cooking time to 3 hours.

Sprinkle with a dash of lemon juice if desired.

Nutrition: Calories: 161; Carbs: 10.2g; Protein: 4.1g; Fat: 13.1g

Chapter 9: Soup and Salad recipes

35.   Carrot soup

Preparation Time: 10 minutes

Cooking Time: 20 minutes

Servings: 4

Ingredients

1 tablespoon olive oil

1 lb. carrots

¼ red onion

½ cup all-purpose flour

¼ tsp salt

¼ tsp pepper

1 can vegetable broth

1 cup heavy cream

Directions

In a saucepan heat olive oil and sauté carrots until tender

Add remaining ingredients to the saucepan and bring to a boil

When all the vegetables are tender transfer to a blender and blend until smooth

Pour soup into bowls, garnish with parsley and serve

Nutrition: calories 123, fat 8g, fiber 2g, carbs 8g, protein 7g

36.   Celery soup

Preparation Time: 10 minutes

Cooking Time: 20 minutes

Servings: 4

Ingredients

1 tablespoon olive oil

¼ red onion

½ cup all-purpose flour

¼ tsp salt

¼ tsp pepper

1 can vegetable broth

1 cup heavy cream

1 cup celery

Directions

In a saucepan heat olive oil and sauté onion until tender

Add remaining ingredients to the saucepan and bring to a boil

When all the vegetables are tender transfer to a blender and blend until smooth

Pour soup into bowls, garnish with parsley and serve

Nutrition: calories 123, fat 8g, fiber 2g, carbs 8g, protein 7g

37.   Creamy Salmon Dill Salad

Preparation Time: 10 minutes

Cooking Time: 10 minutes

Servings: 4

Ingredients:

4 cups filtered water

1 lb. wild salmon

½ avocado, mashed

½ cup fresh dill

2 Tbsp. homemade yogurt (if tolerated)

2 Tbsp. lemon juice

2 Tbsp. fish stock

½ tsp. Celtic sea salt

½ tsp. pepper

Directions:

In a large pot, bring 4 cups of water to a boil. Add the salmon to the pot and boil for about 10-12 minutes, or until the salmon is cooked through.

Remove the salmon from the pot and place in a large bowl. Add the avocado, dill, yogurt (if using), lemon juice, fish stock, salt and pepper.

Mash and mix the ingredients together until everything is combined. Enjoy with a warm mug of homemade stock.

Nutrition: calories 104, fat 8g, fiber 2g, carbs 8g, protein 2.5g

38.   Broccoli Soup

Preparation Time: 10 minutes

Cooking Time: 20 minutes

Servings: 4

Ingredients:

4 cups homemade stock cup broccoli florets

½ yellow onion, chopped 1 clove garlic, chopped

4 tsp. sauerkraut juice

Directions:

Start by adding the broccoli and onion to a large stock pot and bring to a boil.

Reduce to a simmer and cook for 15-20 minutes or until the broccoli and the chopped onion is tender.

Add the chopped garlic, bring to a boil again and then turn off the heat.

Using an immersion blender, blend until smooth and then serve with 1 teaspoon of sauerkraut juice per serving.

Nutrition: calories 123, fat 8g, fiber 2g, carbs 8g, protein 7g

39.   Garden Salad with Oranges and Olives

Preparation Time: 10 minutes

Cooking Time: 15 minutes

Servings: 4

Ingredients:

½ cup red wine vinegar

1 tbsp extra virgin olive oil

1 tbsp finely chopped celery

1 tbsp finely chopped red onion

16 large ripe black olives

2 garlic cloves

2 navel oranges, peeled and segmented

4 boneless, skinless chicken breasts, 4-oz each

4 garlic cloves, minced 8 cups leaf lettuce, washed and dried

Cracked black pepper to taste

Directions:

Prepare the dressing by mixing pepper, celery, onion, olive oil, garlic and vinegar in a small bowl. Whisk well to combine.

Lightly grease grate and preheat grill to high.

Rub chicken with the garlic cloves and discard garlic.

Grill chicken for 5 minutes per side or until cooked through.

Remove from grill and let it stand for 5 minutes before cutting into ½-inch strips.

In 4 serving plates, evenly arrange two cups lettuce, ¼ of the sliced oranges and 4 olives per plate.

Top each plate with ¼ serving of grilled chicken, evenly drizzle with dressing, serve and enjoy.

Nutrition:Calories 259.8Protein: 48.9gCarbs: 12.9gFat: 1.4g

40.　　Lemony Lentil Salad with Salmon

Preparation Time: 20 minutes

Cooking Time: 0 minutes

Servings: 6,

Ingredients:

¼ tsp salt

½ cup chopped red onion

1 cup diced seedless cucumber

1 medium red bell pepper, diced

1/3 cup extra virgin olive oil

1/3 cup fresh dill, chopped

1/3 cup lemon juice

2 15oz cans of lentils

2 7oz cans of salmon, drained and flaked

2 tsp Dijon mustard Pepper to taste

Directions:

In a bowl, mix together, lemon juice, mustard, dill, salt and pepper.

Gradually add the oil, bell pepper, onion, cucumber, salmon flakes and lentils.

Toss to coat evenly.

Nutrition:Calories 349.1Protein: 27.1gCarbs: 35.2gFat: 11.1g

41.   Raw Winter Persimmon Salad

Preparation Time: 20 minutes

Cooking Time: 0 minutes

Servings: 2,

Ingredients:

½ cup coarsely chopped pistachio

½ cup sweet potato, spiralized

1 red bell pepper, diced

1 red bell pepper, julienned

1 ripe fuyu persimmon, diced

1 tbsp chili powder

2 fuyu persimmon, sliced

3 tbsp lime juice

4 cups mixed greens

a pinch of chipotle powder salt to taste

Directions:

In a salad bowl, mix and arrange persimmons, bell pepper and sweet potatoes. Set aside.

In a food processor, puree salt, lime juice, chipotle powder, chili powder, diced persimmon and diced bell pepper until smooth and creamy.

Pour over salad, toss to mix.

Serve and enjoy.

Nutrition:Calories 467.4Fat: 15.4gProtein: 11.3gCarbs: 70.9g

42. Tabbouleh- Arabian Salad

Preparation Time: 20 minutes

Cooking Time: 0 minutes

Servings: 6,

Ingredients:

¼ cup chopped fresh mint

1 2/3 cups boiling water

1 cucumber, peeled, seeded and chopped

1 cup bulgur

1 cup chopped fresh parsley

1 cup chopped green onions

1 tsp salt

1/3 cup lemon juice

1/3 cup olive oil

3 tomatoes, chopped Ground black pepper to taste

Directions:

In a large bowl, mix together boiling water and bulgur. Let soak and set aside for an hour while covered.

After one hour, toss in cucumber, tomatoes, mint, parsley, onions, lemon juice and oil. Then season with black pepper and salt to taste. Toss well and refrigerate for another hour while covered before serving.

Nutrition:Calories 185.5Fat: 13.1gProtein: 4.1g Carbs: 12.8g

Chapter 10: Desserts Recipes

43.   Watermelon Cream

Preparation Time: 15 minutes

Cooking Time: 0 minutes

Servings: 2

Ingredients:

1 pound watermelon, peeled and chopped

1 teaspoon vanilla extract

1 cup heavy cream

1 teaspoon lime juice

2 tablespoons stevia

Directions:

In a blender, combine the watermelon with the cream and the rest of the ingredients, pulse well, divide into cups and keep in the fridge for 15 minutes before serving.

Nutrition: Calories 122 Fat 5.7 Fiber 3.2 Carbs 5.3 Protein 0.4

44. Grapes Stew

Preparation Time: 10 minutes

Cooking Time: 10 minutes

Servings: 4

Ingredients:

2/3 cup stevia

1 tablespoon olive oil

1/3 cup coconut water

1 teaspoon vanilla extract

1 teaspoon lemon zest, grated

2 cup red grapes, halved

Directions:

Heat up a pan with the water over medium heat, add the oil, stevia and the rest of the ingredients, toss, simmer for 10 minutes, divide into cups and serve.

Nutrition: Calories 122 Fat 3.7 Fiber 1.2 Carbs 2.3 Protein 0.4

45.   Cold Lemon Squares

Preparation Time: 30 minutes

Cooking Time: 0 minutes

Servings: 4

Ingredients:

1 cup avocado oil+ a drizzle

2 bananas, peeled and chopped

1 tablespoon honey ¼ cup lemon juice

A pinch of lemon zest, grated

Directions:

In your food processor, mix the bananas with the rest of the ingredients, pulse well and spread on the bottom of a pan greased with a drizzle of oil.

Introduce in the fridge for 30 minutes, slice into squares and serve.

Nutrition:Calories 136 Fat 11.2 Fiber 0.2 Carbs 7 Protein 1.1

46. Chocolate Cake with Chocolate Frosting

Preparation Time: 25 minutes

Cooking Time: 55 minutes

Servings: 12

Ingredients

½ cup cocoa powder

1 ½ cup gluten-free flour

4 eggs, at room temperature

1 cup butter, softened

2 teaspoon vanilla extract

1 teaspoon baking powder

A 23 cm cake tin

1 ¼ cup white sugar

A pinch of salt

For Chocolate Frosting

3 ½ tablespoon butter

½ cup dark chocolate

4 tablespoon water

¾ cup icing sugar

Optional: Sprinkles or decorative hearts (FODMAP's)

Directions

For Chocolate Cake:

Line the baking tin with baking parchment; lightly grease the sides and pre-heat your oven to 350 F in advance.

Put the sugar and butter in a bowl; mix well until light & fluffy.

Slowly add the eggs; don't forget to mix after each addition. Add in the vanilla extract; mix again.

Mix the flour with baking powder, cocoa powder & salt in a separate bowl. Slowly add this mixture to the sugar-butter mixture; continue to mix the ingredients.

Pour the prepared batter into the baking tin & bake in the preheated oven until a toothpick comes out clean, for 55 to 60 minutes.

Let the cake to cool for 15 minutes in the tin and then remove & put on a wire rack to completely cool.

For Chocolate Frosting

Heat the chocolate au bain-marie until completely melted by hanging a glass bowl in a pan filled with hot water.

Melt the chocolate over low heat. When the chocolate has melted; turn the heat off & add the butter. Give everything a good stir until the butter has melted completely.

Slowly add the icing sugar & stirring constantly. Slowly add the water (tablespoons) & stir until you get smooth frosting.

Pour the prepared frosting on top of the baked cake. Immediately put some decorations over the frosting; set aside and let them set.

Nutrition: calories 200, fat 8g, fiber 2g, carbs 8g, protein 6g

47.   **Mixed Berry Crumble**

Preparation Time: 15 minutes

Cooking Time: 30 minutes

Servings: 6

Ingredients

¼ teaspoon baking powder

1-pound mixed berries

¼ cup shredded coconut

½ cup plain flour, gluten-free

4 tablespoon maple syrup

½ teaspoon vanilla essence

Juice of 1 lemon, fresh

¼ cup rolled oats

2 tablespoon raw sugar

¼ cup coconut oil

Directions

Preheat your oven to 405 F in advance. In the meantime; place the berries with lemon juice, maple syrup & vanilla in a small-sized pot. Bring everything together to a simmer & let cook for a couple of minutes, until the juices thicken. Immediately remove the pot from heat; set aside.

Place the flour with oats, coconut, baking powder, raw sugar & coconut oil in a large, mixing bowl; mix until the mixture resembles breadcrumbs, on a low speed.

Evenly spoon the prepared berries mixture into six small ramekins and then top with the crumble topping. Arrange them on a baking tray & bake in the preheated oven until golden on top, for 15 to 20 minutes.

Serve warm with a dairy free ice-cream.

Nutrition: calories 256, fat 8g, fiber 2g, carbs 16g, protein 23g

48.   Peanut Butter Chocolate Chip Cookies

Preparation Time: 15 minutes

Cooking Time: 30 minutes

Servings: 7

Ingredients:

1 cup of natural creamy peanut butter

¾ cup of unsweetened dairy-free dark chocolate chips

1 egg

1 tsp. molasses

1 tsp. pure vanilla extract

1 tsp. baking powder (aluminum-free & gluten-free)

Directions:

Preheat the oven to 350 degrees Fahrenheit, and line a baking sheet with parchment paper.

Add the egg, vanilla and molasses to a mixing bowl and whisk.

Add the remaining ingredients, and stir to combine.

Fill a small ice-cream scoop with dough, level off any excess on the edge of the bowl and drop it onto the parchment lined baking sheet. Gently press down to flatten.

Bake for 10-12 minutes or until the edges are golden brown.

Nutrition: calories 210, fat 14g, fiber 5g, carbs 8g, protein 3g

49.   Star Sugar Cookies

Preparation Time: 15 minutes

Cooking Time: 30 minutes

Servings: 5

Ingredients:

2 cups of blanched almond flour

1 egg

½ cup of coconut palm sugar

1 Tbsp. coconut oil

1 tsp. pure vanilla extract

1 tsp. baking powder (aluminum-free & gluten-free)

Directions:

Start by preheating the oven to 350 degrees Fahrenheit, and line a baking sheet with parchment paper.

Add all ingredients to a food processor and process until the dough comes together.

Roll the dough out with a rolling pin and use a star (or other shape) cookie cutter to cut out 12 stars. Place each star onto the parchment paper gently.

Bake for 8-10 minutes.

Allow to cool before enjoying.

Nutrition: calories 175, fat 28g, fiber 2g, carbs 3g, protein 4g

50.   Brownies

Preparation Time: 15 minutes

Cooking Time: 20 minutes

Servings: 4

Ingredients:

1 cup of unsweetened almond butter

½ cup of raw unsweetened cocoa powder

1 egg

½ cup of pure maple syrup

2 Tbsp. unsweetened coconut butter

1 tsp. pure vanilla extract

1 tsp. baking soda

Fresh mint leaves for serving (optional)

Directions:

Preheat the oven to 350 degrees Fahrenheit, and grease a 9-inch brownie pan with coconut oil.

Add all the ingredients to a food processor and process until smooth.

Pour into the greased baking pan and bake for 20-25 minutes or until a toothpick inserted into the center comes out clean.

Allow to cool before slicing into brownie bites.

Nutrition: calories 345, fat 24g, fiber 2g, carbs 8g, protein 33g

Conclusion

Autism, ADHD, and related issues can be devastating, and it is understandable that dad and mom could want to do something they can to assist their kids. However, the GAPS eating regimen calls for an excellent, ongoing dedication—it's not for the faint of coronary heart, neither is it the best weight loss program for a own family it is acquainted with grabbing meals at the run. Some people sense they've benefited from the GAPS eating regimen, although those reports are anecdotal.

According to its inventor, Dr. Natasha Campbell-McBride, this two-part temporary health regimen promotes healing of the gut, flushes out toxins, and strengthens the immune system. She believes it cured her son of autism and is also good for a wide range of other disorders. Skeptics point out that there is no objective evidence thus far to back up her claims, although research on the GAPS diet is underway at Virginia Commonwealth University.

A list of recommended foods is included in this Guide. However, please note that not all GAPS-recommended foods are immediately digestible. For example, as healthy as they are, leafy greens may be very hard on a compromised system. By starting with only the most digestible items, such as well-cooked, non-fibrous vegetables in meat broth, one's gut begins to heal and rebuild, allowing for the reintroduction of raw produce. I recommend that a person move through the steps in the order presented in this Guide: one to three months preparing for GAPS, approximately one month of Full GAPS, then Intro, then at least 18–24 months on Full GAPS before testing additional foods.

This elimination eating regimen is extremely restrictive for lengthy periods of time, making it very hard to paste to. It may be mainly dangerous for the exact population it's supposed for — susceptible young humans. If you're inquisitive about attempting it, are looking for assist and assist from a healthcare provider who can ensure you're assembly your nutritional needs.